Eternal Youth

UNLOCKING THE SECRET TO HEALTH AND VITALITY

Karen Lyric

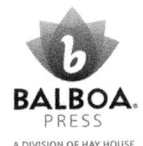

BALBOA.
PRESS
A DIVISION OF HAY HOUSE

Copyright © 2014 Karen Lyric.

All rights reserved. No part of this book may be used or reproduced by any means, graphic, electronic, or mechanical, including photocopying, recording, taping or by any information storage retrieval system without the written permission of the publisher except in the case of brief quotations embodied in critical articles and reviews.

Balboa Press books may be ordered through booksellers or by contacting:

Balboa Press
A Division of Hay House
1663 Liberty Drive
Bloomington, IN 47403
www.balboapress.com
1 (877) 407-4847

Because of the dynamic nature of the Internet, any web addresses or links contained in this book may have changed since publication and may no longer be valid. The views expressed in this work are solely those of the author and do not necessarily reflect the views of the publisher, and the publisher hereby disclaims any responsibility for them.

The author of this book does not dispense medical advice or prescribe the use of any technique as a form of treatment for physical, emotional, or medical problems without the advice of a physician, either directly or indirectly. The intent of the author is only to offer information of a general nature to help you in your quest for emotional and spiritual well-being. In the event you use any of the information in this book for yourself, which is your constitutional right, the author and the publisher assume no responsibility for your actions.

Any people depicted in stock imagery provided by Thinkstock are models, and such images are being used for illustrative purposes only.
Certain stock imagery © Thinkstock.

Printed in the United States of America.

ISBN: 978-1-4525-1862-6 (sc)
ISBN: 978-1-4525-1863-3 (e)

Library of Congress Control Number: 2014912461

Balboa Press rev. date: 9/25/2014

DEDICATION

For everyone seeking health and vitality in their lives. May you live young forever.

CONTENTS

Preface ix
Introduction xi

Chapter 1 - Living in Balance 1
Chapter 2 - Remembering Who You Are 5
Chapter 3 - Finding Youthfulness from Within 9
Chapter 4 - Releasing Negativity from Your Life 13
Chapter 5 - Forgiving Yourself and Others 18
Chapter 6 - Living in the Moment 22
Chapter 7 - Finding Peace 25
Chapter 8 - Having No Regrets 29
Chapter 9 - Loving Yourself 35
Chapter 10 - Being Prepared 41
Chapter 11 - Taking Time for Yourself 45
Chapter 12 - Going with the Flow 49
Chapter 13 - Aging and Your Mind 55
Chapter 14 - Living Your Dream 60

Conclusion 65
About the Author 69

PREFACE

The book you are about to read is a tool for personal transformation. It is a means to assist you in becoming more self-aware. Becoming more conscious and aware of yourself propels you in the direction you are meant to go.

Many people live below their level of consciousness, which leads to confusion and potential errors in their lives. When you choose to live more consciously, you will see the bigger picture and make choices that are in alignment with your true inner self.

I wrote this book in order to assist you to become more aware and apply that awareness to decision making in your daily life. My intention is not to transform you completely but to give you the tools to make choices for yourself.

We live in a world that is very distracting and overwhelming at times. Sometimes people have such bad experiences they shut down and retreat deep within themselves. This results in them shutting off new experiences and they begin to waste away.

Life is meant to be lived. This book will help you do that. If you have suffered in this lifetime, you have the ability to overcome the experience. Life is just that—experience. It is meant to continuously move and flow throughout your lifetime.

We are all aware of the phrase "wasted life". Have you ever stopped to think what that really means? There is no such thing as a wasted life. Life is precious and is a gift we have all been given. It is the gift of experience, and we are all allowed to choose for ourselves how we want to unwrap it.

Most people never live their lives to their upmost potential. But that does not mean it was a waste of time. The point is to remember that you have a choice whether to live or not and how to create what you want to experience. It is that simple. You must give time and attention to yourself and those around you. Always look for signs and clues of where to go next.

Think of your life as a grand symphony where you are both the composer and conductor. Life truly is a stage and you are the star. It is time to start acting like one.

INTRODUCTION

Do you ever wonder why people grow old? Many people would say that it is in our biology, and we simply cannot help it. Others believe that we have no control over our own bodies or our aging process. What if I told you that you do have control and that you can direct your body and mind to stay young forever? Is this true or is it just an expression of a wish or a desire to stay young? Perhaps it is a bit of both.

Inevitably our bodies will age, and we will die. However, the *rate* at which our bodies will age can be influenced by our minds. The evidence is all around us. If you were to place ten people in a line who were all the same age, it is likely that those people would not all look the same. Some would look younger and some older. Is this due to some random event? Does aging simply happen? Are we are at the mercy of our genetic make up or is there something more? Is there something we can do to preserve ourselves in such a way that we look more youthful and vibrant than our chronological age? I say there most definitely is.

There is a lot of information in society today that talks about health and how to stay young. So how is this book going to be different? Why would you waste your time reading yet another person's opinion on how to take care of yourself? Well, this book is different. It will help you discover your own unique personal combination to unlocking the secret of staying young forever. No single formula will work for everyone. What may keep someone else looking young and vibrant may do the exact opposite for another and cause them to age even quicker. Personal choice and diversity has to be taken into account when creating the right plan for you.

This book will teach you how to find your own youthfulness. It will help you to be more in tune with your own individual needs and to find your own personal fountain of youth. Looking and feeling young is a gift that can be had by everyone who chooses it. You do not have to grow old before your very eyes until one day you wake up and do not even recognize yourself in the mirror. There are natural alternatives to staying young besides having to artificially alter your body or its chemistry.

The human body is more capable than we give it credit for. The best thing you can do for yourself today in this moment is to believe that it is possible to stay young forever. Now, this does not mean that you will continue to look or feel exactly the same from the time you are born until the time you die. What it means is that you are in control of how you will look and feel. If you want to stay youthful, it is time to start taking control of your own destiny. If you do not want to become old, then it is in your personal power to do this for yourself. If you are able to suspend all of your beliefs around growing old and can be open to new concepts about how your mind and body can work together to create the image you want for yourself, then you are well on your way to eternal youth.

This book will be able to help you know and understand who you are as a person. Without self-awareness, you cannot influence your body or its processes. The key to understanding the self is being open to whatever information or truth lies within. You must be able to take the bad with the good in order to uncover the truth of your being. The negative aspects of yourself are important, too, and are just as deserving of study as your positive aspects.

Many people age too quickly because they are not integrated and have separated out the undesirable aspects of themselves. The constant inner struggle of these aspects wanting to be recognized creates undue stress on the biology, which in turn causes our bodies to break down at a much faster rate. Aging can be simple or complex, but what it is *not* is something that is out of our control. Do not listen to those people who will tell you that the only way to stay young is to use artificial means. I am living proof that a person with enough self-awareness and a belief system that aging is an option can and will look far younger than her years. It only takes a little bit of effort and time, but the results will most certainly be worth it.

If you already look and feel older than you want, there is still hope. You *can* look younger and almost magically turn back the clock. If you can believe in yourself and your ability to do this, you will be amazed at the results. This book will offer you an easy step-by-step guide to being as young and healthy as you can be. The only obstacle in your way is *you*! The question is, are *you* willing to overcome it?

Chapter One

LIVING IN BALANCE

The key to staying young and vibrant is to allow the time and space necessary to recharge and refresh yourself. Many people are too distracted by outside influences and lose sight of themselves. In order to keep looking and feeling great, you need to make time to get in touch with who you really are. Living in balance means living a life that is right for you. It is not giving away too much of yourself or taking too much from others. It is having the awareness to know when to go out and be with others and when it is time to be alone with yourself.

Many people are not comfortable with being alone and may try to avoid it altogether. But this only leads to a lack of awareness of self and a lack of balance in your life. In order to discover what your specific needs are you must first learn what they are not. Many people realize their true selves simply by the process of elimination. In other words, we learn who we are by first learning what we are not. I am sure we have all had the experience of trying to be someone other than ourselves. Remember how much effort that took? Pretending to be someone or something we are not can add years to our physical appearance.

Stress is the number one cause of aging in the world today. It is everywhere and difficult to avoid entirely. However, there is a lot that we are capable of and much we can do to decrease the amount of stress in our daily lives.

One of the main things we can control is ourselves and that will be the focus of this book. Learning to know yourself will allow you to create a life that is balanced, open, and flowing. By living in this space most of the time you can create an image that is youthful, vibrant, and healthy.

Have you ever been told by someone that you look tired? Looking tired is more than just merely lack of sleep. How many times have you actually had your seven or eight hours of sleep yet woke up exhausted and looking as though you hadn't slept at all? How does this happen? The answer is stress. When you are experiencing stress in your life or a lack of balance, your entire being struggles to correct yourself. If your waking mind doesn't make it happen, then your unconscious sleeping mind will. Unfortunately, when you are asleep you do not have the full awareness needed in order to make the corrections and bring yourself back to your centre. It is much more efficient to do this consciously, and the results will be much quicker.

So how does an individual maintain a balanced and virtually stress-free existence? It is not easy, but it is most definitely achievable. It takes time and effort to be balanced and whole; no magic potion or pill will make it so. Praying will not make it happen either. Only action can bring about the required changes. You can achieve this in as little as ten minutes a day. But those ten minutes must be devoted entirely to you alone. There can be no distractions or outside influences. It has to be only you.

So now you are probably wondering what it is that you are supposed to be doing in those ten minutes. Do you meditate, stretch, breathe, or think? Do you turn on your favorite relaxing music or try to figure out the innermost workings of your mind? The answer is none of these.

What you need to do with those ten minutes is simply be with yourself, completely and entirely. I know this probably sounds too simple but hardly anyone actually does this. You may think you have, but most likely you have not. Being with yourself in the manner that I am describing here means being with yourself fully. It's not about selecting the part that you want to be with and screening out what you don't want. It is about fully accepting yourself, the positive and the negative, and allowing yourself to experience that.

For example, pretend that you had a bad day—you became very upset and angry. Later, you directed that negative attitude towards someone that you loved or cared for. In an instant you felt guilty about doing this but then quickly buried that feeling because you did not want to feel that way. You said nothing and did nothing to remedy your actions.

If you were to do this ten-minute exercise you would re-experience that moment again. It would rise to the surface of your consciousness wanting to be looked at. The reason it would find its way back to you is because you need to accept that part of you that treated another individual in a way that was less than desirable. You need to accept responsibility and then release your feelings of guilt or regret for having done that. If you do not, that experience will stay with you and continue to struggle within you, even if it is buried in your unconscious mind.

The point I am trying to make here is that we have all said or done things that we regretted or that we considered to be negative, yet how many of us took the time to resolve this experience within ourselves? I would guess practically none. Just because we are able to sweep these experiences under the rug, so to speak, does not mean that we should. Every time we do this to ourselves we are unknowingly causing more stress in our inner state. Eventually, this stress becomes more noticeable in our outward appearance. In other words, we age at a more rapid pace.

Now, I have not done any scientific experiments in this regard but I have been watching people throughout my whole life. It is obvious to me that those people who age quicker than others certainly had their fair share of stress. There is an expression that when a person looks older than their years that they have led a hard life. What does that mean? Obviously we have some understanding that stress and aging are related. But there is no real evidence about how much they are related. I believe that these two concepts are very closely related, so much so that if you are able to bring yourself into balance and eliminate the unnecessary stress in your life it will be like uncovering your own secret fountain of youth.

Could it really be that simple? I say it is. If you take the time to know yourself and bring your life into balance your body will reflect that. In later chapters, I will discuss how to balance yourself and your life in a way that will create in you a more youthful appearance.

But for now, I want you to take some time to discover ways that you can do this. Before you read the next chapter I want you to take ten minutes and simply do nothing other than to stay awake and observe your inner state. Do just that; then we will talk about the significance of this exercise in the next chapter.

Chapter Two

REMEMBERING WHO YOU ARE

We are all living in a very fast paced and distracting world. We are over stimulated and do not have enough quiet time for ourselves. Sometimes we are so busy doing things for other people that we literally forget who we are. When we allow ourselves to be so distracted by outer things, we lose sight of our own needs and desires. Many of us struggle to maintain this balance between others and ourselves. It is time to realize the importance of not doing this.

Being out of balance leads to many different outcomes. For example, if we do not have an inner awareness of our self and our state of being it is quite easy to run ourselves into the ground and over work our bodies. Not leaving enough time to rest and refresh ourselves takes a toll on both our physical and mental bodies. The end result can be premature aging.

Many researchers have found evidence to support that sleep is the number one form of relaxation we have in our lives. Sleep repairs and refreshes our bodies. Yet many of us continue to ignore this and try to function on as little sleep as possible. If you are tired, then rest. It is as simple as that. Everything else can wait. You are the most important person in your life. If you do not take care of yourself properly, you will age before your time.

Getting a good night sleep is a simple way to keep ourselves young, healthy, and refreshed. But this is only one of many things that we can do. In the previous chapter we discussed a technique in which you sit with yourself for ten minutes and allow time for connection and awareness of your inner state. Remember what that felt like.

If you have not done anything like this before, it may not have been easy. After only a few seconds you probably became distracted by outside influences. It is not easy to sit with yourself and only focus within. Many variables (including our own minds) will intervene to cause us to look away.

During this exercise it is important to keep re-focusing back to the task at hand. If you find that you are distracted, that is okay. Whenever you notice this happening, just start over and keep trying. The more you practice, the better you will get at it. It is like any new activity that you try for the first time. You cannot expect yourself to be an expert right away. You need to build up to it. If you can do even one minute of this exercise, you will feel much better about yourself.

So by now many of you may be wondering what the point of this ten-minute exercise is. Why should you take precious minutes out of your busy day to simply sit with yourself? It is simply to teach you to realize that the center of your existence is within you. You do not exist outside of yourself. The main focus of who you are is on the inside. Many people may be disturbed by this thought because they have spent so much of their lives looking outwards to define who they are. Just because you have lived your whole life this way until now does not mean you cannot change the way you look at things. All of the accomplishments and relationships you have had throughout your lifetime are important, but they do not define who you really are. The definition of who you are lies within; if you do not take the time to look inward, you will never really understand yourself. So you see, those ten minutes are very important: they are the gateway to your unconscious. Giving yourself the time and space to look inwards will unlock the key to your real identity.

Many people tend to mistake their personality for their identity. I think there is a relationship between the two, but one does not completely define the other. Our personality is something that we create from the time we are born until we die. It is a work in progress and can be changed to suit whatever situation we are in. Our personality is an aspect of our total being but does not completely represent our true self.

So how do we discover our true self? We begin by working at it. We take the time to sit with ourselves and go within to see what is really happening under the surface of our being. When we cut out all of the distractions and outside stimuli of our world and are left with ourselves, only then are we given the opportunity to find the truth. Looking for this truth is the best way to unlock the real you. Sadly, many people do not take the time to do this. They walk around day to day not knowing what is really going on within themselves.

Also, many people purposely ignore their inner state because they are afraid to know themselves. They are afraid that they will not like what they see. It is normal to have these fears but you should not let it deter you from finding out who you really are.

We live in a world of polarity meaning both positive and negative aspects exist. All humans on this earth have experienced or expressed both of these. However, society has set a standard that positive aspects of individuals are sought after and considered better than the negative ones. Naturally this leads to a belief that having negative aspects are less than desirable. As a result, people will reject or hide these aspects. The end result is having an imbalance where only positive aspects are allowed expression.

But what happens to these negative aspects? If we do not allow them to be seen where do they go? The truth is they do not go anywhere. They are alive and well living within you. The reason why you do not pay attention to them is because you have trained your mind and consciousness to ignore them. This is neither healthy nor functional.

I believe people age more quickly than they need to because they do not take the time to allow these negative aspects of themselves to come forward. When we do not like or accept parts of ourselves, we live in a constant state of imbalance and tension—we are stressed out. As we all know, stress can cause a variety of problems: sickness, fatigue, and mental anguish. That is why it is so important to do this exercise. By allowing yourself ten minutes a day to go within and experience whatever you see, you give yourself the opportunity to become aware of who you really are inside.

Once you do this exercise and become more acquainted with your true self, there may be some aspects—most likely the negative ones—that you do not want to face or do not know what to do with. In later chapters we will look at strategies that you can use to help you deal with this dilemma.

For now, continue doing this exercise and practice keeping your focus on your inner state for as long as possible. Once you are able to hold your focus inwardly you will be on the right path to discovering who you really are.

Chapter Three

FINDING YOUTHFULNESS FROM WITHIN

Remember a moment in time when you were very young and go back to it in your mind. Bring up as much detail as possible and the surroundings you lived in. Feel who you were in that moment. Pay particular attention to your sense of youthfulness and your energy level. Young people have a natural abundance of energy; they feel vibrant and almost glow. Most people attribute this state to chronological age. I do not believe this to be completely true. Certainly your age is a factor, but it is only one of many that contribute to the overall sense of youthfulness.

    Youthfulness can be created naturally and from within yourself. It exists not only on the outside, but on the inside. It is a state of mind as well as a state of physical being. When you tapped into the remembrance of who you were at a younger point in your life were you able to catch the feeling or the essence of that youthfulness? If you were able to remember that feeling, what is to stop you from creating this for yourself in this moment? Remembering a point in your life is another form of bringing the past into the now. If an individual has this capacity—and all of us do—it is possible to stay young forever. Wouldn't you agree?

You may say that sure, it's great to remember but I still look old and tired. However, this exercise of remembrance is only the beginning. It is only to show that you have the power to create your inner state. If you choose to be youthful on the inside, this will eventually radiate outwards and you will reclaim that youthful glow you once had.

Aging is partially in your mind and your mind is what creates your reality. If you have a choice to think and feel old or young, which would you choose? So many people just accept the fact that getting old is the natural progression for humans to take. Who says you need to agree with this philosophy?

Personally, I do not want to get old. It does not look like much fun. I have been able to retain my sense of youthfulness, both inwardly and outwardly, simply because I choose this for myself.

I can remember being five years old and thinking to myself that I never wanted to grow old. It disturbed me to see older people, tired and spent and looking as if their very life force was being sucked out of them. In that moment I told myself that I did not want to ever become that way. I decided that as long as I was alive on this earth I wanted to stay young and healthy. There was no other option as far as I was concerned. I simply chose to stay young.

Now, obviously there have been some physical changes and certainly I look older than five, but overall, I have kept the same appearance throughout my adulthood. I have a few fine lines but nothing to indicate my true biological age. If I were to compare myself to others of similar age, there is a remarkable difference. You, too, can do this naturally and simply by *believing* you can be young, and it will be so.

Stepping out of the mass belief system is not an easy task. It took me many years to train myself not to believe what everyone else does. Aging is only one of the many belief systems that I have had to turn away from. I am here to tell you that it can be done. Every day that you wake up in the morning you are faced with a choice. You choose each day, even each moment of that day, to believe what you want. You can either continue to believe what the majority of society believes—that you will continue to grow old and depreciate, both physically and mentally, until you die—or that you can try something new.

You can wake up in the morning and tell yourself that today is a new day, and you no longer believe that you have to grow old. You tell yourself that today is the day you start to turn back the clock and regain that lost, youthful energy that once came so naturally to you. I guarantee that if you tell yourself this each day upon rising that you will start to notice a difference. It may be very subtle at first, but then it will continue to grow and before you know it, you will begin to feel more energized.

Your inner state of being is an important factor in determining your outward appearance. For example, if you are very angry or depressed, what do you see when you look in the mirror? Do you look like your usual self or has your appearance changed? When I am upset and look in the mirror I seem more tired and older than usual. Sometimes I would think I was imagining it, but then I started to notice it with other people as well. Negative feelings are reflected in your appearance. So much so that other people can see it as well. However, you can control your inner state to reflect and influence your outward appearance.

Every day when I wake up I choose to believe that I will not age, or, at least it will be the minimum amount of aging humanly possible. Every day I choose to believe that I will be youthful and energetic because why would I consciously choose to be old and tired? Every day I wake up I celebrate my youthfulness and choose to be healthy and vibrant. I live in a reality where aging is an option. Do I live in denial? Some would say yes. But does it matter? I feel and look my best. How can there be anything wrong with that?

When I see people who are tired and old, I feel sad for them because I know that they can live differently if they so choose. You can start living young again at any time—right now. It is only natural to be skeptical but do not let this prevent you from trying something different. Your belief system is very powerful—much more than you can ever imagine. It is time to start tapping in to that power.

I am living proof that by choosing your belief system you can play an active part in your own aging process. You can start living younger any time you choose. It is entirely up to you. We all have the ability to look and feel our best. Don't you think it is time to start doing this for yourself?

In the remaining chapters you will find some specific exercises on how to change your belief system and clear out some of the obstacles to allowing your youthfulness to return. In the meantime, simply be open to the possibility that what I have said could be true. Wake up in the morning and start each day believing that you could be younger if you choose. This is an important beginning to regaining your youthfulness and changing your belief systems once and for all. Remember, inside you is the key to being young. All you have to do is use it.

Chapter Four

RELEASING NEGATIVITY FROM YOUR LIFE

As I mentioned earlier, one of the key factors that contributes to premature aging is the amount of accumulated stress and negativity that is contained within you. Many people hoard their experiences and refuse to let go of them. It does not matter whether these experiences are happy or sad; they just choose to hang on.

When we were children, our parents and mentors didn't always teach us how to let go of things. Perhaps that is because there is an unspoken belief in society today that it is not appropriate to do so. Many people believe that their experiences define who they are, and that by letting go of them they might lose a part of themselves.

When you hang on to past experiences you prevent yourself from moving forward into the future. Hanging on to the old, leaves no room for the new to manifest. Letting go of the past contains the key that will open the door to your youthfulness.

Getting older is a fact of life. Gaining wisdom is a choice. If you were to find knowledge that could help you stay young far longer than most, wouldn't you want to explore this further? Many people are afraid of letting go of the past because it contains experiences that they want to remember and re-live at will. Letting go of these experiences does not mean forgetting about them; it only means you are putting them in their rightful place and keeping yourself more current and fresh. Letting go of the past enables you to live in the now.

By living in the moment, you can utilize the tremendous amount of energy available to you throughout your day. Living in the past burdens you by taking much of that energy away.

Your past experiences naturally want to be put away, but your mind and your being are so powerful that they can override your own natural processes. Hanging on to things will not allow you the freedom to live fully and, more importantly, will cause undue stress on your physical body. This translates into premature aging.

Let me tell you a story about a young girl who grew up in a very dysfunctional family. There was a lot of conflict between family members, and nothing ever was resolved. These experiences continued to happen on a regular basis. Over time all family members, but especially the little girl, started to live in the darkness of their past.

Each individual began to deteriorate and age quite rapidly. Everyone was tired and moody with no energy left over at the end of the day. Even though they would sleep for hours, many of them would wake up already tired. This was a very sad family indeed. The little girl was especially sad.

One day a stranger approached the little girl and asked how she was. Out of habit, she lied and said she was fine. But the stranger knew better. He could see the sadness in her eyes and hear it in her voice. He leaned in and whispered to the girl that the key to happiness in this world was forgiveness. The little girl had heard of forgiveness, but her parents had never taught her how to forgive.

The little girl looked up at the stranger and asked, "What does that mean?"

The stranger replied, "Just let things go."

At that point the little girl began to cry because she realized that the reason she was so sad and distant from others was because the many negative experiences in her life had caused her to simply give up. It was easier to give up her energy and youthfulness than to fight for her true self. At that moment the little girl made a decision to live out the rest of her life free from past experiences. Each day would be a new day. No matter what happened the day before—as good or as awful as it was—she would simply leave it in the past and start each day anew.

I was that little girl. I made that choice because I realized that my only chance of creating happiness for myself would have to come in the present moment, the *now* moment. I have learned from my past experiences, but I use the wisdom I gained in the *now*. I do not go back into the past for it is gone. I can remember it if I wish but quite honestly I really don't want to. The minute I start reliving the past is the minute I stop living in the *now*. Doing that would affect how I create my future.

To stay in the *now* moment you must first make a choice to let go. Take a moment to decide what you will do. If you want to move forward and make changes in your life read on. If not, I will be waiting for you if you change your mind.

The most important thing you can do to facilitate letting the past go is to simply make a decision to do it. Believe me, it works. Once you have made that decision the energy of your life will flow in that direction. You will then attract what you need in order to be successful.

One of the simplest ways to learn this is to use positive affirmations. What this means is that if you self-talk yourself into believing you want to let go, you will be motivated to do it. You might start by saying every night when you go to bed, "I choose to let go of my day." That is it. You just need to state it that way. Details and specifics are not important. What is important is your intent. Make a choice to let the events of the day go, and then you will be successful. As you sleep, you will naturally let go of things and your memories will be filed accordingly.

Alternatively, if you go to bed without affirming this, your sleep would be quite different. You will wake up continuing on from the day before. However, if you take the time to simply state your intention to let the day go, you will be fresh to start again when you wake up in the morning. Try this for a week and see if you notice a difference in your mood and how you start each day. Once you are in the habit of doing this, you will no longer have to say the affirmation because it will have become automatic and a way of life that is very natural, requiring little effort. Once you are in the flow of this you can start to let go of the past that you are still hanging on to. It is better to start with the *now* because it is important to first stop your habit of not letting go. Then you will not accumulate any more baggage.

The next exercise is also simple, but the effect will be quite strong. I want you to pick a memory of something that you consider to be negative or unpleasant. Once you have found that memory write down two or three feelings about it. For example-anger, sadness, disappointment, fear, and so on. After that, write down feelings opposite to those. When you are finished imagine putting all those feelings into a big pot stirring them together. Then throw away the pot. Throw it as far as you can imagine.

Now sit with yourself for a minute and feel what is going on inside you. Do you feel relieved? Do you feel lighter? Do you feel freedom? If you have done this exercise properly, it will help you release past experiences that you are hanging onto.

The important thing to remember is that it can work if you want it to. The past does not have to continue to prevent you from moving forward. We have all had negative experiences in this life that we were not happy with, but we do not have to continually re-live them and be at the mercy of their destructiveness. Past negative experiences do not have to influence our future. How will you choose to live?

Chapter Five

FORGIVING YOURSELF AND OTHERS

In the previous chapter we talked about learning to let go of the past. Forgiveness is similar. It is also a form of letting go but it is more specific to a certain type of feeling. I want you to remember a time when you were hurt by someone. What did you feel in that moment? Were you sad, angry, afraid, or unbalanced? When another person says or does something to us that we feel is negative or uncalled for, we form an experience with that person that binds us together. That experience becomes locked into our psyche. Unless we make a purposeful attempt to resolve it, it will remain with us.

Forgiveness is the mechanism by which you can release yourself from that experience. Unfortunately, this does not happen often. It is more likely that when another person harms us we hang on to that experience and think that if we do not forgive that person we are punishing them. But, did you know that the only person you are truly punishing is yourself?

When you hang on to those negative experiences and do not forgive, you are causing undo pain and suffering to yourself. Many people believe that by forgiving others we let them off too easy, or that people who forgive others are weak. That is untrue.

Have you ever watched a movie where an individual went to another who had harmed him and told him that he forgave him? Did you see the release and sense of peace that occurred? That is forgiveness. It is a way to let go of unnecessary stress and tension that only serves to hold you back from moving more freely into the future. When we hang on to old situations, hold grudges against others, and refuse to forgive them, we are only hurting ourselves. Forgiving more often and more completely is an important factor in keeping ourselves young, vibrant, and healthy.

Learning to forgive is not an easy task, but it does get easier with practice. Sometimes we set limits on when to forgive. For example, many of us will not forgive others until they apologize and appear remorseful for their actions. Sure, it is nice to have an apology, but what if it never comes? If you do not forgive others, you hang on to the negative feeling of the act itself. Most often the other person is the least affected by the situation. Sometimes the other person will not even be aware that he upset you.

The important thing is that when you are upset about another you are the one who has to forgive. Forgiveness is not about who is right or who is wrong. Forgiveness is simply allowing resolution to a situation. It is making a decision to let go and move forward. It is acknowledging that yes, you were hurt, but you are not going to hang on to the pain and cause yourself needless suffering past the point of the experience.

The key in life to staying healthy and happy is to always move through each experience moment to moment and to not hang on to the past. As I mentioned earlier, you cannot live in the past because it is not healthy or natural. The present moment exists for a reason; that reason is to live in it. Just because your mind can exist in the past or the future does not mean you should. The past and future are a nice place to visit but your primary point of reference should always be in the *now*. To live otherwise will only wear you down. You must let go and forgive others in order to be your best. You will feel much happier, lighter, and be able to live more freely if you do.

Learning to forgive others is very important, but so is also learning to forgive yourselves. We are much too hard on ourselves as humans and hold such high standards that we set ourselves up for failure on a continual basis. We always think we are more capable of doing what we can than we actually are. You can only be who you are. Certainly it is good to have goals and want to create changes for yourself, but in this moment you are who you are. You must learn to accept that and, most importantly, learn to forgive yourself.

I want you to close your eyes and breathe deeply for a minute. Become as relaxed as possible and try to clear your mind. When you are in a relaxed space, remember something about yourself that you do not like. It can be anything: a body image; an act you were involved with; or something you wanted to accomplish but didn't. The important thing is to remember an instance in your life that caused you to be disappointed or upset with yourself.

Once you have that memory in your mind feel the impact of that judgment you had on yourself. Feel the way it has settled into your body, your mind, and your identity. Feel how pervasive it has become within the totality of your being. Then, reverse into that moment and re-live it. For example, suppose that you wanted to complete a task but did not have the time or became distracted and did not do it. Imagine that instead of criticizing yourself you forgave yourself and understood it was okay to do this. Tell yourself that no matter what happened, you are worthy of love, and you are willing to let go of the expectation that you originally placed on yourself. Sit with that feeling for a moment, and then slowly open your eyes. Can you feel the difference now? Do you feel lighter and happier, perhaps even relieved? This is the power of forgiveness.

All you need to do is recognize those moments in time when you labeled yourself to be less than deserving of your love and then correct it. Allow yourself to go back to that moment of perfection within yourself that we are all born with.

We can only do so much as humans, and we all make mistakes. We can do as much harm to ourselves as we can do to others. It is important for your well-being and the well-being of those around you, to continue to move forward and let go of those times in your life that were not favorable or did not live up to your standards. Forgiving yourself will allow you the space within yourself to be perfect as you already are.

So many of us forget how beautiful we really are. A negative self-image can destroy us from the inside out. If we allow our inner beauty to shine, our outward appearance will grow to reflect that as well. If you are kind and forgiving to both yourself and others, you will have a natural glow and radiance that cannot be duplicated. Practicing forgiveness in your daily life will eventually become a habit. Once you have mastered this task, you will be well on your way to eternal youth.

Chapter Six

LIVING IN THE MOMENT

A growing movement in society today is telling people to live in the present moment. You can find many books and discussions on the topic, yet do we really fully understand what this means? I think there is still some confusion, which is why I want to take the time to talk about this further. The very simplest definition of living in the moment is to live fully in yourself. If you can do this, then you are truly in the present. But what does this mean? It means you are living with the you contained in the *now*. It does not mean you are focused on the past or the future self; only the present version of you is important.

Existing fully in the *now* allows you to function at your optimum potential. More energy flows into your being. The things that sap your energy are eliminated. You will feel better, look better, and accomplish so much more when you can do this for yourself.

Training yourself to live in the moment is not as hard as it sounds. There are various techniques you can use throughout the day to help you focus. For the next day or two simply observe your thoughts. Take notice of what you are giving attention to. For example, do you tend to think more about the past or the future? Most of us exist in one domain or the other. Certainly there are moments when you are present in the *now*, but probably you are focused on either the past or future.

Once you have observed where you comfort zone is, ask yourself these questions: "Why do I choose to be focused on the past or present?" "What causes me to leave my present awareness and drift away from the present moment?"

Really think about these questions. Write down whatever answers come to you. Do not judge your responses. (Your mind commonly does this.) Just let the answers flow to you freely, openly, honestly and without hesitation. Let it be natural and uninhibited. When you have your answers, create some solutions that will assist you to move through these barriers. Every answer that you uncover is a barrier to living in the present moment. It is important to address this as soon as possible so that you can change.

I will give you an example of a potential barrier to living in the present moment. When I did this exercise, I found that I was always trying to be a better person. I wanted to be smarter, in better physical shape, and financially well-off. These attributes were important to me. I spent quite a bit of my day focusing on how I could create a better future for myself.

Now don't get me wrong, there is nothing the matter with having goals or wanting to create things in the future. This is natural. If there were no focus on the future whatsoever then not much change would be happening day to day.

What I am talking about here is something different. Constantly focusing on the future and wanting things to be different is not appreciating who I am right now. Indeed, it is difficult to accept myself in this moment without wanting something in my life to be different. It takes a lot of practice to learn to live in the moment and actually be happy about it.

We all want our lives to be different or better, but how many of us can truly say that we are happy now no matter what? How many of us can actually be ourselves in the moment and not want to change anything? Very few, I bet. For those who have achieved this, congratulations! This is one of the most important attributes a person can have.

The present moment contains all of the energy and wisdom you could ever want. So much power lies in the moment, yet when the day ends we are always left feeling depleted and tired. Feeling exhausted is an important indicator that you are not living in the *now*.

Living in the moment means you have enough energy throughout the day from start to finish, so that when you do go to bed at night you feel relaxed not stressed out. So much of our stress comes from our own minds when we do not allow ourselves to just be in the moment. We worry about things we have not done and things we have done. No worries exist in the present moment.

Life poses many challenges for us and leads us into the future. The key is to balance. If you want to live at your highest potential, keep reminding yourself throughout the day to be present. Try to catch your mind when it wanders into the past or future. Do not let your mind dictate where to focus your thoughts. You have the ability to be in charge of your own reality. Start doing this for yourself. When you live in the moment and are living to the fullest potential of your being, you will be naturally energized, youthful, and vibrant. Existing in the past or the future will only serve to deplete you and cause undue stress, which is an important factor in premature aging. How will you choose to live? I definitely pick the present moment. How about you?

Chapter Seven

FINDING PEACE

We are currently living in a hectic, fast-paced world where there is little time for rest or relaxation. Constantly bombarded with stimuli, we rarely take the time to release all of the pent-up energy and stress from our day. We go to bed wound up and anxious from our day and do not allow ourselves to release these feelings and experiences. How are we to find peace within ourselves when we are living a life that does not allow for this to happen? The answer is simple—we must make it happen. We as individuals are the only people who can help us to relax and live a peaceful existence. Many different strategies and outlets are available for your use. What is important is to find the ones that work for you.

Take a moment right now and close your eyes. Imagine a time when you felt at peace with yourself and the world around you. It can be as simple as a brief moment in time, or a relaxing vacation you had. If something does not come immediately to mind, imagine something that would give you a sense of peace in your life right now.

When I do this exercise I find peace by creating within myself a safe and healthy space with no outside influences. The sense of peace comes from an understanding that everything is okay and perfect in this precious moment. Even though this is an imagined state that I create for myself, it brings me a true feeling of peace.

Your mind and imagination create feelings. Are you able to remember a feeling without any thought attached to it? There are probably very few, if any. The point I am trying to make here is that where thoughts go, feelings and energy flow. If you want to be more peaceful in your life, all you have to do is think that feeling into existence and it will be so.

You may be skeptical here because I am sure that you have tried to change your emotional state at one time or another but were not very successful. Many of us have wanted to be less sad or angry but felt powerless to change our condition. The reason we were not able to do this in the past is because our belief systems prevented us from doing so. They are so powerful that they can create or destroy the very nature of our being if we allow them to.

Society generally dictates what to believe, but as individuals, we also play a part in creating our belief systems. We have more personal power than ever before and can use this power to create our own reality. For example, if you had a stressful day that left you tired and irritable, you do not have to feel that way all evening. You have the power to change your emotional state to one of being peaceful, happy, and content. All you have to do is tell yourself how you want to feel and what emotional state you want to be in. I know this may sound crazy, but it really does work.

Over the next week I want you to become aware of a point in time when you were feeling upset. When you have time to be alone, dwell on what triggered that feeling. What caused you to react in that way? Once you have pinpointed the true cause of the feeling, acknowledge the feeling and then simply choose to release it. Release the trigger and the resulting emotion simultaneously. Once you have released them, you will be left with a sense of peace and resolution. It is very subtle, but you will feel it. Congratulations! You have just successfully influenced and created your own emotional state. You see, it is not that hard. Just start out slowly and simply. Before you know it, you will become a natural expert at it.

Now, a word of caution. These exercises are not aimed at helping you to escape or avoid your daily experiences. You still need to process your feelings and give attention to them as they come up. These exercises are meant to assist you in transforming feelings that you have already experienced, not dismiss or avoid those that are still seeking expression. We all need to be accountable for our experiences in life and the resulting emotions that accompany them. However, you do not need to be at the mercy of your emotions or allow them to dominate your existence. Emotions are a key ingredient in what makes us human. We need to allow them expression, but we do not have to let them run amuck in our lives. We can decide for ourselves when we have had enough.

Having a sense of peace in your life is crucial to your health and well-being. Without peace you will always be in a chronic state of stress. Stress ages us prematurely and causes our bodies to break down at a faster rate. When it comes to wanting to look and feel younger, stress is not our friend. It works against everything we want for ourselves. Stress may be inevitable at times and must be experienced, but it does not have to be chronic or endless. If we manage our stress and allow ourselves the space and opportunity to create peace, we will be well on our way to being our youthful and vibrant.

It is important for you to find out what brings a sense of peace to your world. Creating peace in your mind is one way to achieve this, but there are many other ways in which to do this. A relaxing walk, a warm bath, a good book, or a night out on the town, are all examples that may work for you. Physical exercise is an excellent way for the body to dispel stress from itself. You need to find a routine that works best for you.

It is not so important what you do to relax and find peace but to find something that works, and works well. Also, remember that you can change over time. What you might find relaxing one day will not necessarily bring about the same results the next. Keep current and keep changing with what you need. Peace is a very important factor in our health and well-being. You need to create this for yourselves and teach others you care about to do it as well.

The more peaceful we are within ourselves, the more peaceful our planet will become. We all want peace in this world, it can start as simply as with you. Be an example and others will follow. Finding peace in your lives and in your hearts will result in all of us living happier and healthier lives. Caring enough for yourself to do this is an important beginning. That is what futures are created from.

Chapter Eight

HAVING NO REGRETS

At one time or another, all of us have regretted leaving something behind in the past that we wish could be in our present. A part of us, no matter how small, is still hanging on to something from the past. Usually this something prevents us from moving forward in our lives. This could be a past love that we still regret not having a relationship with, or a career path that we chose over another. It could be pretty much anything we can think of that, when we had a choice to make at a point in our lives, we chose something else. Each day we are faced with many decisions from the very simple to the extremely complex. When we choose one outcome over another occasionally some residual thoughts or feelings remain. Unless these are resolved, they will cause us undo stress.

Try and remember a time in your life when you were faced with an important decision that entailed picking from at least two different options or paths. Remember how it felt to go through the process of having to make the decision. Now remember the point at which you finally decided which option to choose. In that moment you may have not been completely certain about your decision, but you were willing to move forward with it and give up the alternative, whatever that may have been.

Pretend that instead of making the decision that you did, you picked the other path instead. Feel the potential of that decision and the impact it would have on your life today. Imagine what the result would have been if you had gone in another direction rather than the one you originally chose for yourself.

I can guarantee that the other option would have had a different outcome than the one you picked. You would have met different people and had different opportunities. Your life, as you know it, would not even exist. This is important to know.

When you are faced with a decision, the option you choose will change your life. The ones you don't pick would have changed you as well but in a different fashion. The point I am trying to make here is that you can live only one life when you pick one path over another. There may be similarities, but they are not completely compatible. If they were, you would not have been put in a position to choose in the first place. You could have had either path.

When you are choosing between two people for a relationship, it is clearer that you cannot have both (although some may think they would like this). You can only have one wife or one husband. So if you were faced with a decision whether to be with one person or another, it is impossible to have these two paths at once. Yet how many of us reminisce about our past loves and what could have been? How many of us think "what if" or try to imagine a life with another? Do you think this is only imagination or is it having a real impact on your life today? I believe that it does.

Remembering the past and imagining a life other than the one you have currently created for yourself confuses your being. Your biology, your sense of self, and your emotions are all connected to your mind. When you allow your mind to wander into the realm of imagination, you are creating something real. The mind is an interesting part of being human, there are so many unknowns as to the power that it truly has over us. But, enough research is available to indicate that the mind does influence us more than we realize. For example, athletes use the power of their minds and imaginations to improve their performances. Results show that this really does work. Children use their minds to imagine their futures. That is what creation is made of. If we did not use our minds to imagine a future for ourselves, what do you think would happen? My guess is probably not very much. The future would come as planned, but there would not be much in it.

The mind is a very important tool in creating our reality. When we use it to imagine potentials or situations that are not going to be created, it is a waste of our time. It is not even entertaining. Most of the time when we use our minds to remember the past or try to imagine what our lives would have been like if we had gone in a different direction we are bringing a level of negativity to that experience. We remember in a sad or regretful way. If we are truly happy in our present lives, why would we even want to imagine or remember something that we originally decided we did not want? It doesn't make a lot of sense, does it?

Many times when we try to recreate the past we are attempting to escape from our present reality. We are not choosing to live in the moment or be who we are. Instead, we are wasting our time. If you are not happy in the present moment and want to change your life, you must use your mind and the power of your imagination to create something that you want for yourself.

Going back into the past will never help you move forward into the future. It may be a nice place to visit some time, but it really has no bearing on what is happening with you right now and most definitely has no value in creating your future. The future is born out of what you think and feel in this moment, not the past. If you are hanging on to past issues, this will influence your current state of being, which in turn will influence your future. Remembering old potentials or paths that may have been options in the past is not healthy or functional, unless you are thinking about actually doing something about it. For example, if you regretted not finishing a school program and decided to go to back to complete it, you would be making good use of your time. But, simply thinking about how you really wanted to finish school but never did and still don't plan on it, is a waste of your time. Do you see the difference?

Let go of your old regrets. It is time to start living in the *now* and get on with your life. If you are not happy, use the resources you have to start creating a future for yourself in which you can be happy. Forget all those people and opportunities you once had that are no longer available in your present reality. Life is so very short, and opportunities always present themselves to us. If you are too busy dwelling on the past, you will miss what is right in front of you in this moment.

Regrets in the form of unfinished business in our lives continually drain us of our energy throughout our day. If you want to be young, healthy and vibrant, you have to start acting in a way that promotes or allows that to happen.

In order to help you move away from the past and let go of any regrets you may have, I am going to give you a short affirmation. Use this affirmation when you find yourself drifting into the past and feeling those old regrets coming to the surface. It is important to have some self awareness around this because if you cannot even recognize if or when it is happening, you will not be able to make the changes necessary to let them go.

When you feel you are in that space and starting to remember something from the past that you continue to have regrets about, take a deep breath and bring yourself as completely into the present moment as you can. An easy way to do this is to simply observe your breath as it flows naturally in and out of your body. If you do this for 10 or 15 seconds, you will be able to be more focused.

Once you are feeling more present, say to yourself: "My life is here and now. I have made many choices, which have led me to this point. I understand that there are different decisions I could have made, but in the moment when I had the choice to make them, I chose differently. I have no regrets about these decisions. I completely release any resistance I may have to letting them go. I am who I am in this moment. I cannot recreate my past. The only path I have to create for myself comes from this present moment. I choose to move forward from this point only. The past is the past, and I am now ready to lay it to rest."

This is a powerful exercise. If you truly understand and believe the nature of these words, you will be successful in letting go of any unfinished business you may have as a result of past regrets and making decisions. That will always be the case because all of us are faced with making so many decisions in life.

Choice is an important part of being human, but so is being okay with what we decide. When we let go of the past, we open ourselves to being fully in the present and enjoying the path that we have chosen for ourselves. Living freely in the present moment enables us to better create the future we want for ourselves as well. It is important to remember that when we let go of anything that is holding us back—including our regrets—we become lighter, more youthful, and have more clarity in what we want to create for ourselves.

So many of us feel stuck in our lives because we do not let the past go. In turn, this gives us a bleak outlook on our future. It is no wonder that we live in the past because it is the only place we feel that we have to go. A vicious cycle is created when you continue to live in the past and recreate it. It is time to break that cycle. The tools I have presented to you in this chapter will assist you in reaching this goal. Remember, you have the power of your mind and your imagination to create the future that you want. All you have to do is try.

Chapter Nine

LOVING YOURSELF

Do you ever wonder why people are so sad and lonely? What is the cause of all of this? The world is filled with so many people, yet everyone at one point or another in his life feels completely alone. No matter how many people you are close to or who love you very much, if you do not first love yourself, none of this will mean anything to you.

Now, there is more public awareness of the topic of self-love in society today. Everyone who has heard of this concept knows what it means. Or do they? What is love anyway? So many people have tried to define it, yet they always seem to come up short. There are so many different meanings for love and so many classifications or types that people are left feeling lost in their understanding of it.

Love is not complicated. It is a simple emotion that occurs naturally between two people who care about each other. What makes the concept of love so difficult to understand is how people have distorted the true meaning of it.

So let's start with an exercise where we will uncover our own individual beliefs about what love means to ourselves. Close your eyes and breathe deeply for a minute or two. Try to clear your mind and relax your body as much as possible. When you are feeling relaxed and centered in your mind, think about love and feel what it really means to you. When you have a clear picture of your belief, write it down on a piece of paper. Include everything you can think of.

Once you have completed the list, go over it and add anything you feel you may have left out. The list could be quite short or very long. It doesn't matter about the length: just make sure you have as much written down as possible. When you have finished this list, crumple up your paper and throw it in the garbage. This may be difficult for some of you, but it is very important that you do this. Once you have thrown away your list, come back, and we will talk about the point of this exercise.

Many of you are probably wondering why I asked you to do this exercise. You are probably thinking: "What is the point of doing this if I am not going to keep a list of all of the hard work I just did trying to understand the meaning of love?"

The simple explanation is that there is no definition of true love. It cannot be defined. It is beyond human words or comprehension. The human understanding of love is limited to the human mind which is not capable of fully understanding and defining love. I wanted you to do this exercise to show you that all the examples and feelings that you came up with during the exercise are not representative of the true meaning of love.

We have all had experiences in life where we thought we felt love, but this is only a glimpse of the true nature of it. Love is so much more than many of us realize. We are all familiar with different expressions of love, but so much more about it can be discovered.

One of the ways in which we can experience more fully the concept of love is to practice on ourselves. It is easier to start with ourselves than to try to love others. Many people think it is the opposite, that it is easier to love someone else but this is an illusion. We are really only loving others in a limited fashion so it only appears easier. Many of us love conditionally and situationally. We also love others related to our ability to love ourselves. Many of us do not even know what that means. Can you imagine how much love there would be in the world if we all started with ourselves first? It would be almost unbelievable to even conceive of this happening, but it is possible.

Self-love is the most powerful and real love you can ever experience. Once you have tapped into this feeling, you will never want to live without it again. Self-love fills the holes inside you. It takes away that feeling of emptiness and separation that so many in this world struggle with. It allows you to become happier, and healthier, a whole person.

Self-love is reliable and unconditional. It stays with you throughout your entire life and will never leave you. It is the constant companion that you have been searching for. When you have self-love, you can love others more fully and completely. It is the only true love that we can create for ourselves.

Logically then the next question is: what is self-love and how do we create it for ourselves? Defining self-love is simple: it is accepting yourself for who you truly are. It is first knowing yourself and then being okay with what you find. It is the closest thing we can think of when we talk about unconditional love.

We think of unconditional love as the greatest love there is: this is probably the closest definition to love that we can have with our limited human understanding of it. We cannot love another this way if we do not first apply it to ourselves. Loving someone else unconditionally without first loving yourself, is not real. It is an illusion, and like all illusions, they will eventually be exposed for what they are. You must first love yourself, and then you will be able to love others in the same way.

So how do we do this? How do we find it within ourselves to truly accept and love ourselves? This in not an easy task, but it is certainly possible.

The concept of self-love is gaining more publicity these days. As people become more interested in the topic, they are starting to gain an understanding that you must love yourself first before you can really love another. If we could all love ourselves first, there would be far less heart break and sadness in the world. So many people feel the loss of love in their lives, especially when someone they love leaves them. They are left with a big empty space where the love for that person once existed. Why does this happen? How can love be there one minute and then gone the next? That should be our first clue that what we thought was love was not the real thing.

True love is eternal. It has no boundaries and exists whether the person is with us or not. When we lose someone in our life for whom we felt love, our sense of loss and pain is our own neediness. It is not that we have lost love; it is that we have lost someone who was filling a need for us that we were not filling for ourselves. Do you understand the significance of knowing this?

When you truly love someone there is an air of lightness to it. There is a freedom in knowing that you will love that person whether he or she is in your life or not. When you love another with conditions or attachments, you are twisting the concept of love into something else. That is why so many people are confused these days about what love is.

Love has no negativity or attachment. It is a very subtle energy that flows through us and exists in the world for everyone to experience.

But the key is to allow it to move and flow through you. The minute you try to possess it or control it, you turn it into something else. Does this sound familiar?

How many times in your life do you try to control or manipulate the ones you love to become something that you want in order to fulfill your own needs? I am sure it happens quite often. It is a bad habit that we have all been taught from a very young age. It is time to let that go and the best way to start over is to begin with loving yourself.

The first step in learning how to cultivate self-love is to spend time with yourself. Think of this as being similar to how you would date another person. When you are interested in someone and think a relationship is possible, what do you do? You spend time with them in order to get to know them better. It is in these moments that love is created.

The same is true with the experience of self-love. You must first get to know yourself. The only way that is going to happen is if you make time to sit with yourself. Many people are afraid to know themselves and avoid time spent alone, but you must overcome this fear if you want to learn self-love. You do not need to spend hours alone; even 10 or 15 minutes a day would be great. It is the intent to know yourself that will make you successful. If you are sincere about wanting to learn self-love, it most certainly will happen for you.

The easiest way to start this process is to recognize qualities that you like about yourself. Think of one or two things you feel are good qualities and then allow yourself to feel love for yourself as a result. The positive qualities are good place to start with because it is easier to love those types of qualities than the negative ones.

But, the negative ones need love too. Most of us disapprove of our negative qualities, and we judge ourselves harshly for them. But this only creates self-hatred. That is not what this chapter is about.

Feeling love for yourself unconditionally means to love and accept both your positive and negative qualities. This process can be as easy or as complex as you make it. Self-love can be born out of the simplest concept—acceptance of yourself. If you practice self-acceptance, you will naturally create self-love in return.

Perhaps there are barriers in your mind to doing this. At this point it may be helpful for you to process what it is that is blocking you from accepting yourself. In the end, it is really all about your willingness to do this. Practice accepting yourself completely and you will be surprised how fast your feeling of self-love grows. Self-love is contagious. Once you start, it will take on a momentum of its own. Eventually, you will also become more in love with other people in your life. Then you will begin to experience what true love really is.

Love is so important to our existence and well-being. It keeps us healthy and gives us a sense of purpose and belonging in this world. People who feel love will reflect this in their outward appearance as well. In other words, love makes you look good. Love keeps us young, healthy and vibrant. It does not make sense to rely on others for this feeling when we have the ability to create it within ourselves. When you are able to love yourself, you will never be without love again as long as you live. What could be better than that?

Chapter Ten

BEING PREPARED

Many people go through life in a state of uncertainty. They do not trust that their future is safe or friendly. Many carry with them unnecessary fear, which is the ultimate breeding ground for stress. Does it really make any sense to fear the unknown? If you were to look back on your life and examine how your future unfolded, how many instances of actual distress are there? For the average person, there are not many. Certainly there are some people who do have negative experiences that will impact them tremendously. It will take a lot of inner strength and will to overcome this.

But I am not talking about these people. They are the exceptions rather than the rule. The majority of us go through life with relative ease. So why do we constantly fear the unknown? Why do we allow ourselves to be fearful and stressed out over events that have not yet occurred and perhaps never will? It is because it has become a habit. We are following in the footsteps of our ancestors, and it is time to start over.

If we have a choice to welcome the future and the unknown without fear, then why don't we do this? It is time to believe that our future can be, and generally is, friendly. We do have some influence over what our future holds so what it comes down to is this: do we trust ourselves enough to believe that we can create the future that we want? The answer is "yes" and the time to start is now.

When people first inhabited this earth, I can only imagine that there were a lot of unknowns. In the beginning, the focus would have been on survival. Many people did not understand the nature of the world and how it worked. People were most likely in a state of fear because they did not know what their future was going to be. They probably felt victimized and at the mercy of some unknown force. Does this sound familiar?

After many generations and experiences we still hold on to this primal belief system. It is time to let it go. Because we have evolved so much as a species, the element of fear that our ancestors originally possessed is no longer needed.

We all know our world a lot better now and have a greater understanding of how nature works. We have more control than ever before over our future, so why do we still fear it so? It is time to start anew and believe in yourself. It is time to tell yourself that you can trust your decisions and the plans that you make. You are safe in this world and can create exactly what you need or want in order to be successful in this life.

Now, simply allowing yourself to believe that you will be safe and secure in your future is an important step, but it is only one piece of the puzzle. You also need to start believing in yourself. That is the most important thing you can do. Many of us doubt our ability to take care of ourselves. As a result, we rely on others for our safety and well-being. This has got to stop. I am not saying that you should not have support from others because it is fine to have supportive people in your life. The point I am trying to make is that you also need to learn to be self-sufficient. You need to believe and realize that you have the potential to take care of yourself and your own needs. You do not need anyone else to fulfill these needs for you.

For example, in the not so distant past there was a belief that men were supposed to get married and take care of their wives. Men had to financially support the women, and they in turn took care of the house and children. Then, times changed. Women decided they wanted to get out of the house and do different things. Many began careers of their own and found satisfaction in this. The result was a generation of women who were self-reliant. They no longer needed husbands to look after them. They could actually do it on their own.

Yet many women today still hang on to this old belief system. This belief has been so ingrained in us from past generations that it is almost encoded in our very DNA. So while a part of us believes that we can take care of ourselves, another historic part is continually working against us. A part in all of us still believes that we are not able to take care of ourselves because that is what history has taught us. But times have changed and this belief system is now sorely outdated.

Tell yourself out loud that you no longer are willing to accept the belief that you are not able to provide for yourself and fulfill your own needs. Renounce that old belief and allow the new one to become present in your reality. It is time to own your own power and realize that any human on this planet—man or woman—has the same ability and potential to take care of himself.

Exceptions will always exist, of course, especially for those with limited physical or mental capacity. But the average person should start looking after himself and his own needs. Become self-fulfilled and self-reliant. Think of how much happier and confident you will become going into the future if you truly believe that you have the strength and the power to create your future exactly how you want it to be.

You are not at the mercy of unknown elements. You are not waiting for some other person to come and rescue you from the world. You are your own best friend and your greatest asset. If you can capture the essence of what I am saying here, you will have no reason to fear your future any longer. When you let go of the fear, you will lessen the amount of unnecessary stress that you are creating.

Try to live in the moment as much as you can. All too often we spend too much time focusing on a future that has yet to be created. By giving too much energy to this, we are drained so much that we are too tired to live in the moment today.

Creating the future should be effortless in the sense that we probably only need one tenth of the energy that we are currently allotting to it. Having some focus and direction for our future is necessary, but only enough to create the potential for it to happen. The remainder of our time and energy should be here and now. That is where our true self lives and where our optimum potential lies. It is time to let go of our unnecessary fears and live freely and confidently. The less fear we have, the less stress we create, and the more energetic and youthful we become. Just try to live this way and watch for yourself what the results are. I am sure you will be pleased.

Chapter Eleven

TAKING TIME FOR YOURSELF

When we are living in such a fast-paced and hectic world, it is important to slow down every once in a while and take care of ourselves. We are so used to taking care of other people, whether it is our families or the work that we do. But how many of us take the time to do that for ourselves? There is a growing awareness in society today that we do need to focus on our own needs, at least once in a while, in order to stay healthy and balanced. However, we are usually at the bottom of the list. All too often, by the end of the day, we are usually the ones who get brushed aside. It is time to start making ourselves a priority and put ourselves at the top of the list where we truly belong.

Self-care can mean many different things. It could include making sure you get enough sleep or that you are eating a healthy, balanced diet. It could mean finding some form of relaxation or engaging in physical exercise. There are so many things that we could do for ourselves. Many of them really don't take too much of our time. The trick is to make this a priority and get it done. If we don't, then the stress in our lives will continue to build until one day, we will not be able to live at our optimum or fullest capacity that we are capable of.

Self-care is so important because it is the one thing that we can do for ourselves, which we do not need anyone else to do for us. We have the power to control our own bodies. We can make our own decisions around health and well-being. We can no longer blame others for our state of mind and state of being when we possess the tools and resources necessary for us to be healthy.

People who have had a stressful day and do not find a way to release that feeling will eventually become burnt out in their daily lives. The accumulation of stress may not noticeable all of the time. It has a way of sneaking up on us. Many of us do not even realize that we are stressed out. Many of us think that to be irritable and tired is just what life is like. This is not true. We all have the potential to live long, healthy, and youthful lives that are full of energy. We do not have to grow old and tired just because we are alive. Being alive and living our lives can be very enjoyable. Unfortunately, so many people have come to believe that life is stressful, we simply grow old and die, and that this is what people do.

However, every once in a while you see an older person who has an abundance of energy and is enjoying life to the fullest. These people stand out. We take notice of them for they are very few and far between. But how sad and unfortunate is that? Why is it the exception and not the rule to live life in your older years just as you would when you were younger? It is obviously possible and you can see from some people that they are doing it. So what is stopping you from living this way? Have you simply given up and accepted the beliefs of others so that the very act of being alive literally sucks the life and energy right out of you?

I say, "No more." It is time to change your belief systems and start living differently. You do not have to become tired and grow old before your time. Stress happens. We encounter difficult situations on a daily basis. Our jobs are stressful, our families are stressful, the food we eat is contaminated with pesticides and the air we breathe is full of impurities and toxins. So what? Do we continue to use these situations as an excuse to wither and die, or do we actually do something about it to change ourselves? It can be done, and it is being done by a select group of people in this very moment.

If you take the time to really take care of yourself, you will see a significant change in your mental, emotional and physical well-being. If you give yourself only one half an hour a day to pay attention to yourself and release the stress you have accumulated throughout your day, you will naturally become more youthful and vibrant. I cannot emphasize enough how important this is for you. Stress kills you slowly and silently. It diminishes your quality of life, and it poisons your physical body.

Why do we continue to allow ourselves to reach this point when we have the power to prevent this from happening? Do not let yourself be overcome by your experiences in life. Do not let yourself come home at the end of the day and fall into bed with no energy left in your body. If you are this depleted, you have not successfully let go of anything.

Tiredness is the first sign of unresolved stress in your life. Sometimes we are tired because we are sick or lacking sleep, but most of the time we are tired because of stress. Do not blame others for your stress in life because if you do, you lose the power to change your situation. If you believe that others are the cause of your stressful experiences, you will have no way to change your life. You will always be at the mercy and control of outside influences. This needs to stop.

If you can accept the fact that you—and only you—are responsible for your thoughts, feelings and actions, you will have the power to change how you relate to the world and those around you. This is very important to know because it can help you improve the quality of your life in so many ways.

In this world where we live with many others, we will always likely encounter someone who does not agree with us. Differences are okay. But, we need to be prepared and have the awareness to know when we are allowing these conflicts of interest to get the better of us. Stress is an inevitable part of life, but that doesn't mean that we have to become subservient to it. We can learn many things from being under stress. Sometimes it even motivates us to act. But it should be a transient quality, not an enduring one. Once the stressful situation has passed then we should let go of the feeling, not hang on to it as many of us do.

You need to find an outlet that works for you so that you can release the stress that you have experienced throughout your day. It is very important to come up with a wellness plan, one that works for you. Read about various health and relaxation practices and see which techniques work best for you. Keep doing this until it becomes an integral part of your daily life.

If you can commit to just half an hour a day, you will have added many years to your life and given yourself a much healthier and youthful appearance. Life is not perfect, but we have the power within ourselves to learn to be okay with that. Make the commitment to change your life, you will be greatly rewarded. It certainly has worked for me.

Chapter Twelve

GOING WITH THE FLOW

A lot of stress in our lives is the result of not getting what we want or living the life we want to live. Many of us are continuously unhappy about our lives, but instead of doing anything to change it, we sit in it and are stressed out by it. How many hours of your life have you wasted worrying about something that you have no control over? An example of this is bad weather. It is very common for people to complain and be stressed out when the weather is not pleasant. Does this make any sense? You cannot control the weather, yet so many people act and complain about it.

It is time to take a personal inventory of your life and stop being stressed out by those things that simply cannot be changed. Certainly there are many things that can be, and I would strongly encourage you to pursue this. But what I am talking about here are those things in your life—especially the outcomes or experiences in the past—that you cannot change.

So many of us waste our time, focus, and energy on these things. We are all guilty at times of even wanting to remember our suffering. Sometimes when we do this we actually feel better about it. But taking pleasure in past negative experiences does not make any sense. Recalling these experiences and refusing to let the memory go will age you prematurely and cause so much unnecessary stress in your life. Why would you choose this for yourself?

It is time to let go and go with the flow. When you hang on to the past or try to recall memories of things that have happened, you are disrupting the natural flow of the present moment. Every time you use your mind and put your thoughts elsewhere, you are interfering with the natural flow of your life. It is important to stay current because if you continue to live the way most of us have been living, this will take years of quality living away from you.

Stress kills. This is a proven scientific fact, yet many of us fail to heed this warning. We think that exercising or eating right will take the stress away, but this is not going to get to the core issue: why we are stressed out in the first place. The only way to know why each of us experiences stress is to go within ourselves and take a personal inventory of those experiences and situations that we label as stressful. This is the starting point we all need to have. Once we can identify the root causes of why we become stressed out, we can go to work at eliminating them once and for all.

The first important step in doing this is to allow time to be with yourself. When you are alone, the focus is completely on you. There are no outside influences and no external people to blame for your inner state. It is only you.

Many of us avoid being alone with ourselves because we are afraid. We are afraid that if we take a closer look and try to find out who we really are that maybe we will not like what we see. A lot of truth lies behind this fear because many of us really do not like ourselves, not completely. If you can think of someone or something in your life that you think is negative or distasteful, then chances are you feel the same way about some part of yourself as well. This is called mirroring and simply means that many of us project our own inner rejection and dislike of ourselves onto others. In other words, what we dislike about another is really a mirror of something we do not like about ourselves. All you have to do is pay a little more attention to yourself to know what is going on in your personal reality.

Pause here and do a short exercise. Think of a person in your life who has recently caused you to feel negative about something. Pick a situation that you can vividly remember how upset you were with this person. Once you have caught the feeling, turn the situation around completely. Imagine that you are now the person who is acting in a hurtful way towards somebody else in your life. Become that person and express yourself in exactly the same way.

How does it feel to be on the other end of things? Many of you may feel anger or regret or even shame at having reacted that way or treated someone so badly. Chances are that some time in your life you were that person, and you never had the chance to really resolve the conflict within you. It is hard to think positively about ourselves when we act in ways that are hurtful or negative towards others, especially towards people we love. Certainly, many of us do apologize for our actions, but how many of us take the time to apologize to ourselves? It may seem silly but all of have an inner critic that judges us harshly for these things. This inner critic is very self-righteous and not very forgiving. It is this aspect of ourselves that keeps us in a state of self-hatred and stands in the way of our self-acceptance.

It is okay to make mistakes in this world. All of us have said or done something in our lives towards another or ourselves that was not very nice. But, it is time to move on and let it go. Whenever you hang on to the past, it imprisons you in that time period. There is no flow when you are stuck in the past. You are like a backed up toilet, full of crap that has nowhere to go. It is time to lighten your load and learn how to become more open and flowing in your life, both within yourself and with others. When you can do this for yourself, you will be well on your way to a happier, healthier and more youthful future.

So by now you are probably thinking that this sounds like a good idea, but how do you change the way you have been living all these years? It is easy enough to talk about but how do you actually allow yourself to live in a freer, flowing manner? The best place to start is in your own mind. Your mind controls your reality and your thoughts. Thoughts in turn influence feelings and behavior, so you must go to the source of your suffering, which is contained in your own mind.

The mind is not your enemy, but it can stand in the way of your happiness. It is very bossy and likes to believe that it is always right. In fact, being right is one of the main goals of its survival. In order to retrain your mind to think more positively and be more in the present moment, you have to allow yourself to go back into the past and put to rest, once and for all, those experiences that you have not been able to completely resolve.

Traumatic or unacceptable experiences leave a broken memory. Part of the reason we as humans like to recall past experiences—especially traumatic ones—is that we are looking for resolution and closure. Unfortunately, there are so many wounded people in the world who have their own unresolved issues that we have no real guidance to move forward. We keep telling our tragic stories to others who share similar experiences. As a result, there is little or no movement. It is time to stop doing this. You will always find a sympathetic ear, but this has not served you well up until this point. Complaining about the past does nothing to fix it. In fact, it is like opening an old wound over and over again so that it has no opportunity to heal.

The only way you can find resolution to your past is to do it yourself. Only you can heal yourself, and it must be from the source—your own mind. It is time to realize that you are in control of your own reality and have the power within yourself to change your life and how you choose to live it. It is nice to have someone to support you when times are hard, but it is completely unnecessary to continue to tell your story over and over again. That is not healthy for you or the person who is listening.

Negativity is stressful and not something that you want to have ongoing in your life. Stress has its time and place in this world, but we have accumulated so much of it in our daily lives that it has become incredibly toxic.

It is time to let go of our negative experiences, towards ourselves and others. It is time to start developing a greater awareness of ourselves and what causes us to think and feel negatively about life. When we find the root cause of what makes us think this way, we are well on our way to understanding ourselves better. Once we understand ourselves, we can truly start to live in a healthy and flowing manner.

Nothing is worse than not knowing ourselves yet continuously blaming others for our problems. This makes no sense. If we continue to live our lives in this manner, we will literally start to break down, physically, mentally, emotionally or all three.

Take time in your busy day to sit with yourself and get to know yourself. Look at your past experiences. Find those moments that continue to be a source of stress for you. Once you eliminate past stressful experiences and find those aspects of yourself that have caused you to think negatively about yourself and others, you will be on your way to truly managing your stress in the best way possible. Being in the moment and flowing day to day takes practice, but practice makes perfect, and that is exactly what we all are.

Chapter Thirteen

AGING AND YOUR MIND

The relationship between mind and body has been studied for many years. A growing body of research shows how these two aspects of your being are interconnected. You cannot favor one over the other. You must learn to balance the two. Yet many of us continue to allow our minds to dominate our reality. If this is the case, maybe it is time to take a personal self-inventory of what you are using your mind for. In other words, if you are living mostly through the awareness of your mind, what are you thinking and saying to yourself throughout the day? This is what I would call self-talk. For most of the day, we talk to ourselves in our minds. Some of us even talk out loud. The point is that something is always going on in our minds because the mind likes to make noise and be noticed. A quiet mind can be achieved through meditative practices and other relaxation methods.

So what is it that we have so much to talk about to ourselves during the day? The majority of our thoughts are not positive or supportive. I would bet that most of what our minds tell us is negative and self-defeating. Why would this be the case? If we can choose our thoughts, why would we more often than not choose negative ones? The answer is simple: our minds focus on the negative because most of the drama and energy are there.

Our minds are bored when everything is okay and nothing needs to be talked about. A quiet mind is simply boring, and we don't want to be bored. So if our minds want action, then let us give them just that.

But, we still have a choice as to what our thoughts are. Many of us think we are in control of our own minds, but really our minds are controlling us. A lot of what we choose to focus on and think about is from the past and can be considered a repetition or pattern of events. The mind likes to be in control. Since the past has already happened, it is a favorite source of information to tap into. However, the mind tends to wander towards the negative rather than the positive. This is something that we certainly have the ability to change—if we want to.

The first and most important step to controlling your thoughts is to simply become aware of them. For the next two or three days, I want you to conduct an experiment on yourself and simply observe your thinking. The best time to do this is when you are idle and not engaged in conversation with others. It is too distracting at first to start this way, so it is better—at least for now—that you do it when you are alone.

A way to see what others are focusing their thoughts on is to listen in on conversations. You will learn a lot about people and how they think. When I first did this exercise on myself, I was shocked to see how many of my thoughts were organized around negative concepts. I do not consider myself to be a negative person by any means. I generally like to think that my mind is peaceful and balanced. However, when I observed my thoughts for the first time, the amount of negativity was quite noticeable. What I discovered was that I had a habit of focusing on the negatives instead of the positives. I do not remember when this started in my life, and I don't even know why it happened. The important thing I did learn was that I did not want to be thinking so negatively throughout my day, so I made a conscious choice to change my thoughts. It took some time and practice but eventually it did work.

Once I made the decision to stop thinking so negatively, I began to work on changing this. I did this by being more aware of my thoughts and stopping any negative thought processes. There were a lot of them! Even to this day I do experience some negative thoughts. You cannot eliminate them for good. But now I am more balanced, and the tendency for my mind to focus on the negatives has been eliminated.

It is important for you to realize the focus of your thoughts because in order for you to stay young and healthy you need to have a mind that thinks along those lines as well. You won't be healthy and vibrant if your mind continues to send you unhealthy thoughts. You need to coordinate your beliefs around being able to maintain your youthfulness with your mind; otherwise the two will work against each other. The mind is a very powerful tool that creates your reality and your beliefs about yourself and the world you live in. You need to form a conscious working relationship with your own mind so that you can create the best life that you are capable of. One of the best ways to do this is to start talking positively to yourself.

Positive thinking is not a new topic and there are many published books and research in this area. However, there has not been much discussion on how positive thinking can affect your own body. A branch in science, known as psycho-neuro-immunology, describes how the mind influences the body and its chemistry. I am not going to discuss this area in detail, but I would encourage you to look into this for it will help you believe what I am about to say next. Your mind has a great influence on your body and if your mind believes that you are getting older, then you most certainly will.

I know a lot of people who are starting to get older. You would not believe how often I hear people make comments about themselves that are negative and ageist. So many talk about their hair turning grey or thinning, their bodies getting fatter, saggier, less attractive, and their faces getting wrinkled and dry. I hear so much about it, but I am sure that it is only a fraction of what those people are saying to themselves every day. It is no wonder that their body gets the message that they are aging.

Have you ever heard the expression that you are what you eat? I would like to take that one step further and say that you are what you think, literally. Our bodies are made of energy, and our thoughts are the same. The two interact and negative thoughts of growing old and our bodies deteriorating become a reality. When I hear people complain about getting old, I tell them that they are only making matters worse by accelerating their aging process. Certainly our bodies will age over time, but our minds play an important part in the rate of how and when that will take place. Perception goes a long way. It is time to start allowing our minds to work for, not against us.

In my daily reality I do not allow myself to think I am aging. In fact, I tell myself, every day at a conscious level, that I do not want to grow old. I do not want to have saggy wrinkled skin or loss of my senses. I tell myself that whether I am 20 or 50 years old that I am going to look the same and have the same health and vitality that I always did. Why not think this way? What is the alternative? To think that I am going to grow old and die? What fun is that?

Just think of the words and feel the energy behind them. If you choose to be positive and say that you are going to be young, healthy and vibrant, what type of feeling and belief do you get? Alternatively, when you say that you are going to grow old, get fat, become unhealthy and tired and eventually die, what type of energy and feeling do you get from that? I am sure it is quite obvious. The positive stream of thought nourishes your body and mind into a healthy state while the other more negative stream of thought moves your body and mind towards deterioration and eventual death. So what will you now choose to focus on?

Your body is constantly changing and renewing itself in many ways. When you do decide to change your thoughts, your body will respond. Positive thinking may not create a noticeable miracle or take 50 years off your life, but it will rejuvenate you and allow your body to become more youthful and vibrant. There are no limits on what you can believe. If your mind has to be active and thinking of something, why not steer it more towards the positive rather than the negative? Negative thoughts do not allow your being to live to its full potential. It limits you and what you can achieve for yourself in life.

Being positive and believing in the unbelievable is what dreams are made of. Dreams *can* come true. If you nurture and love yourself from the inside out, you will see a change in yourself. Your body will react positively. We can't all be supermodels, but we can be our personal best. No matter how old you are, it is not too late to change. Believing is the first step. What do you choose?

Chapter Fourteen

LIVING YOUR DREAM

I have spent a lot of time throughout this book discussing how to live your life so that you can retain a youthful, healthy, and vibrant body and mind. Now is the time to start putting that into action. Living life is an opportunity that we seldom make the most of.

When we are young, we seem to live life more fully. We take chances and are adventurous. We like to try new things, meet new people and discover who we are. It is unfortunate that as adults we lose this innate ability to create ourselves and our lives. It is as if when we are older we reach a level of comfort and certainty and then stop growing and changing. We just settle into the life we have created for ourselves and slowly age into our future. Just because we have a career or a family doesn't mean we have to stop living. Life is full of surprises and there is always something new to learn or discover. Let us go back to when we were children and capture the essence of that time period.

Let us tell ourselves that even though we are adults, having routines and responsibilities, it is okay to step out of that once in a while and try something new or different. It can be as simple as listening to different music or seeing a movie that is not in our usual taste. It can be trying a new restaurant or vacation destination. There are so many little things that we can do to take us into a new level of experience. It does not have to be drastic. The main point I am trying to make here is that even though we spend a lot of time in our youth discovering our identity and who we are, our likes and dislikes, there is still room to grow and change within ourselves. Just because we have grown older and wiser does not mean we have reached the end of the road just yet.

Times change and people change. Technological advances occur rapidly these days. Many older people today are missing out on an amazing time in this world. Take the time to learn new things; you will discover a part of yourself that you never even knew existed. Always consider yourself a work in progress.

Change is good. It liberates us from the stagnant flow of life that we all too often tend to become bored with. There is no reason to be bored in this world. There are such a diverse amount of people, culture and experiences that it is not humanly possible to ever know everything that there is. We all exist in such a small slice of the total reality of this world. It is time to start discovering what is truly out there and leave the security and confines of our daily life that we have created up until this point.

Life is short but we make it shorter than it has to be when we stop looking for new experiences and opportunities, for new expressions of ourselves. Let us all become young once again and welcome the sense of personal discovery that once shaped us into who we are now.

Nothing is wrong with what we have become, but we still have a long way to go and many opportunities to discover even greater things about ourselves. Let us be brave and move forward in life with a fresh spirit and a willingness to go beyond what we currently know. Generation gaps exist for this very reason. People become comfortable and then stop learning and growing. This does not need to happen. We all have the same capacity for learning and experiencing no matter what our age, physical ability, or personal situation. Just because we are aging does not mean we have to do it quietly. Youthfulness feeds our souls when we allow the essence of it to stay with us throughout our lives. If you give up on feeling young, you will age too fast. If you tell yourself you are tired and do not have the energy to do anything other than what you are already doing in your daily life, you will live that reality over and over again. When people get stuck in repetition and convince themselves that this is what life really is, they are missing out on so many possible opportunities.

Very few people on this earth ever live out the potentials available to them. We can create new experiences every single day of our lives until we die. It is time to start living life to the fullest. Whatever you can think or dream can become a reality.

But, you must first start by believing it is true. If your belief system does not support the reality that you can change and manifest what you want for yourself, you will never be able to create what you want in your life. It is called self-sabotage, and we have all become experts at it.

We are so beaten down by this world and our past struggles that we think there is nothing left for us in the future. We slowly give up as we get older and just settle into the reality that this is all there is. We need to snap out of this mentality and start anew. We need to first believe we can create our realities and then start imagining the future we want for ourselves.

Everybody has dreams in this world, things that we all want for ourselves. So what is the difference between those people who are able to make their dreams come true and those who don't? The answer is simple: none, except that the people who make their dreams happen wanted it to happen. They believed in themselves and their ability to create what they wanted. They had faith and were motivated. Even in the face of adversity they never gave up. They never became discouraged or allowed others to stand in their way.

To those individuals who want to live beyond the norm, many people say that it is not possible and try to convince them that it won't happen. We are so brainwashed and beaten down by life that we literally don't want others to succeed because if they do, it shows us that we are not living with the same capacity. We need to start living fully and start believing that we can create our own realities. If you put any effort at all into living your dream, you will see results. Be sincere and most of all believe in yourself. Do not rely on others for support or guidance. Be your own person and accept full responsibility for both your successes and your failures. Never give up because the moment you do, you will be settling for less than you truly deserve.

Start by focusing on simple things that you want to have happen in your life, and work from there. Once you become confident in your ability to create the things in your life that you want, you can start doing this on a grander scale. Most people want to start big. This is not very realistic for the majority. Always keep your goal in mind but know that the path to achieving your goal can involve many steps in between.

Life is a work in progress. It will continue to be that way until it is your time to leave this world behind. Live life to the fullest and you will be rewarded. If you become discouraged along the way, take a break and rest. Once you have regained your strength and motivation, continue on. Never give up and never allow your personal setbacks to prevent you from moving forward. You are the author of the wonderful mystery that is your life. What kind of story will you choose to write?

CONCLUSION

By now you have hopefully gained a better understanding of how to promote and create youthfulness in your life. Being young takes some effort, but mostly it takes action on your part. The world can give you many reasons for being stressed out. The tendency to shut down, give up or become bitter is a natural human response. But there is another way to live, and that way has been presented to you throughout this book.

It is time to start living more naturally and more freely than you have ever done before. It is time to regain your youthful sense of adventure and desire to learn new things. Just because you have lived a long life already does not mean you have reached the end of your journey. Your journey in life begins anew each and every day. Your sense of who you are, your identity, can be built upon in each moment until your death. Life is a continuous experience; it will not end until you take your last breath. If you believe in yourself and your ability to wake up each day with an intention to learn something new, it will happen. All you need to do is open your eyes and open your heart to drawing new experiences to you. It may take some practice since you have become used to living a certain way, but it can definitely be achieved.

The most important thing to remember is that you have an abundance of energy within you that is waiting to be generated and expressed. You have the power to create what you want and, most importantly, what you deserve.

Do not allow yourself to be beaten down by your past. Your past was an important part in shaping who you are today, but it is not the end of things. The now is the new beginning that you have been waiting for. It has always existed, but you did not even know it was there until you made a conscious choice to look at it.

Many people wait until they are diagnosed with a terminal illness or experience a tragedy before they make a decision to really start living. Why wait until that moment? All of us will die one day so if we know that day is coming, why not start living more fully now? Nobody wants to think about his own death, but if it will motivate you into taking action, it needs to be mentioned here.

Make a list of things you want to do in this world and then set out to do them. Spend time with people you care about because who knows when they will no longer be in your life. Eat healthy foods, get plenty of sleep and take care of your body as much as you can. You will feel better about doing new things if you feel good first. But, even if your health is failing, there are still opportunities to learn and do new things. Many people in society today have shown that physical or mental limitations can be overcome. We are all more capable than we truly know. It is time to start living up to our full potential.

Life can be a joyous and wondrous adventure, which does not have to stop just because you feel you are getting older. The fountain of youth, contained within all of us, is just waiting to be discovered.

I have shown you the path to get there, but it is now time for you to take control of your own life and do the work necessary to actually create it. We are all on a personal journey in this life and have great opportunities to make lives that we can be proud of.

I hope that all of you reading this book will go forward and start to live life to the fullest so that when it is your time to leave this world you will do so without regret. Take the time to nourish yourself and you will be rewarded. Remember the youthfulness that you have long forgotten and bring it back into the present moment. Feel your youth returning to you as you allow your mind to settle into the now. Release the past and leave the stress behind you. Stress will not feed your youthfulness; it will only take it away from you.

Regain control of your own mind and the way you want to live your life. Be patient with yourself and do not allow others to deter you from your goal. Many will not want to believe that much of what I say is true or relevant, but let me ask you, what have you got to lose? If you take the time to reconcile your past, become more present in the moment, and live life to the fullest, how can you go wrong?

Make those changes that are necessary so that you may once again live young and free, both inwardly and outwardly. Take the time you need to regain your inner sense of self and create whatever you want or need to be happy. Let go of those people and situations that are negative and holding you back from creating what you truly want. Forgive those who have hurt you and, most importantly, forgive yourself. Accept your imperfections and allow yourself to truly express who you really are.

If you accept yourself, you are free to be whom you choose; nobody can take that away from you. You will always encounter some form of negativity in the world, but you have a choice whether or not to internalize it or allow yourself to be affected by it.

You must be strong in yourself to be true to what you believe and not follow the opinions of others. Many people want to conform and be accepted in society, but that mentality is creating a world of actors and illusions. To be genuine and real is the biggest challenge we can face, but the rewards are endless. It would take only a few people to be true to themselves for others to follow.

Be a leader not a follower. Try new things and new ideas. Test things out and see if they ring true for you or not. Most importantly, always keep moving forward and you will eventually reach your goals.

I wish you all of the best on your life journey and hope you will be successful in creating the perfect life that is meant exclusively for you.

ABOUT THE AUTHOR

Karen Lyric has spent the past twenty years working with children and families as a social worker and counsellor. She graduated from the University of Manitoba with a Bachelor of Social Work Degree in 1995 and moved to Vancouver, British Columbia shortly after where she now currently resides.

Karen has a unique combination of both personal and professional experience which she is now passing on to others. She has devoted her life to helping people and has transformed herself into becoming a more healthy, happy and self-aware individual. Her message is intended to help others to do the same.

Notes

Notes

Notes

Notes

Printed in Dunstable, United Kingdom